The Zombie Fitness Manual

Helping the Undead Look Alive

P.J. Hafner

Birchbark Publishing

Publisher's Cataloging in Publication
Hafner, P.J.
The Zombie Fitness Manual / P.J. Hafner
p.   cm.
ISBN-13: 978-0615633220
1. Exercise – fitness   2. Exercise – zombies   I. Title

Contents

Disclaimer

Consult with your physician (leave his/her brain intact, please) before you begin to participate in any workout or exercise program, including exercises in this book. I'm not a medical professional and do not claim to be. I've performed all the activities listed within, and the described exercises have helped me maintain my fitness level. I have confidence in the enclosed exercises and believe they will help you keep in good form and prevent your body from falling apart as you go about your daily activities.

But as required in books of this type, I must state that using the guidelines included in the following pages is done at your own risk.

Introduction

So you're a Zombie now. A new phase of life (or non-life?) that can be exciting, intriguing, and adventurous. A never-ending quest for the bodies of the living, especially those nourishing brains, can be rewarding and satisfying.

But not if you proceed unprepared; leading a life as one of the undead while ill-equipped can be disappointing at best, disastrous at worst. You may find yourself frustrated. Failing to plan and to ready yourself can lead to aimless wandering, constant hunger, and a persistent feeling of coming apart at the seams.

What's that you murmured? You're already falling apart? Uh, well...let's come back to that a little later. Anyway...

Pursuing your newfound passion for brains requires some skills. As competition heats up, you'll want to keep yourself ahead of the curve and increase your success rate in satisfying that never-ending brain urge. To help you attain that goal, this manual outlines some exercises sure to help you get ahead and outcompete your fellow Zombies.

Many of your cohorts will continue to stagger, stumble, lurch, and shuffle. Be different. Don't submit to peer pressure. Rise above and leave the less capable behind. It's all fair in the age of the post-apocalypse.

Ever fall over, and find yourself unable to easily get back up? At times have your prey clutched in your grasp and they simply wiggle away? Endure members of the living, those you seek to conquer, taunting you as they easily evade capture? Have no fear. The power-enhancing motions in this manual will help you rectify those problems.

Just one warning before you begin: This program takes some commitment for you to succeed at it. No feeling sorry for yourself. Stop moaning and take charge. Well, as a Zombie it's natural to moan a little, we understand that. Just make sure the moans are predatory in nature, not ones issued as complaints.

Dig deep. Some of you reading this manual may have previously dug yourself out of the earth to start your new life. So feel confident in the fact that you already have some practice in this area.

To motivate yourself, try to envision the brains you seek. Dream of them, imagine savoring them. They are the Zombie's Holy Grail, after all; know that the regimen in these pages will help get you some. Mmm.

Be aware, though, to acquire more brains, you've got to use your own – whatever's left of it anyway.

But that's part of the benefit of using the methods offered in The Zombie Fitness Manual; you don't even have to operate with a full deck to take them up with success. Give this program even a partial effort, and you'll be able to munch, crunch, and lunch with greater ease and higher frequency. What do you think? Sound doable? It seemed like a moan you just issued, so we'll take that as a *Yes*.

Excellent! Let's get started.

The Warm-Up

Walk It Out

If you have time, start off each fitness training session with a short walk. Lumbering a city block or so often does the trick for most Zombies. This will warm up your muscles and serve as a small workout in and of itself.

For the living, it was long advised that walking would help maintain bone density and prevent osteoporosis. This may or may not provide the same benefit for you; walking's effect on bone health for the undead has yet to be proven. But walking should at the very least get you good and loose for the heavier lifting just ahead. Plus, if you choose to do some energetic arm flailing and moaning, it can be a nice practice session for your hunting endeavors.

Walking is one of the simplest exercises; it requires no equipment aside from a good, supportive pair of shoes. If your footwear has long since deteriorated, see if you can't extract a newer pair off some of the fallen in the areas you trudge through.

Or just kick off the old shoes and try walking the classic and natural way: barefoot. Nothing captures the post-apocalypse spirit like stomping about looking for prey with bare feet. Give it a try.

By and large walking is a lower body exercise, but with a vigorous arm swing your upper half will also get warmed up nicely. With time you could add some resistance, mainly to share the burden of the workout with your upper body. This can be done with hand weights, light dumbbells, or even fist-sized stones you find lying around in the wasteland.

Walk that city block or so at least every other day; this exercise should be done above and beyond your normal seeking of victims. As your walking program progresses, you might find it easier and easier to move at a brisk pace. Soon you should see your pace improving from slow motion to speedy.

Just wait until you see the look on the faces of your prey, as your former stagger turns into a self-assured stride. Surprise! Keep up the walking regimen, and it'll happen.

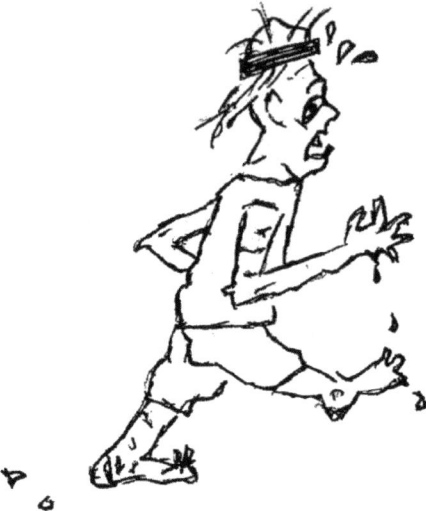

Jump Rope

Here's an old standby for an energizing warmup. When you jump rope, you'll activate many sections of your body, in particular those parts that stay intact. Key areas which may benefit include your hips, lower legs, upper legs, arms and shoulders. Pretty good deal for a single exercise.

Jumping rope as part of a solid exercise routine seems to have went by the wayside over the years, and that's been a mistake. Here are some functional benefits to jumping rope:

- Better capability for leaping and seizing prey that may be climbing up and away.

- Improved skills in bouncing on your toes and maintaining balance when pushed back by a potential victim.

- Stellar ability to jump up and down in celebration of a food conquest with your fellow Zombie tribe members.

- Helpful for effectiveness when stomping on a downed foe.

- Increased lung capacity – this is a great cardiovascular exercise.

- And much, much more.

To proceed, find a piece of discarded rope, twine, or rubber band. The length should be such that when you hold one end of the rope in each hand and stand in the center of the rope, the ends in your hands reach your waist (too short and you'll keep tripping over the rope; too long and you could get tangled up). If the length of the material is just a bit too long, simply adjust your grip as needed. It will be hard to find the exact, optimal length of rope or band; scavengers in the wasteland can't be too particular, after all. Do the best you can.

Holding one end in each hand, simply twirl the rope from the back, over your head, to the front and jump over it as it swings towards your feet. After a few failed tries and enraged yells, see if you can't get a nice rhythm going. Continue until you start getting tired, then call it a day.

If you get bored with the forward direction, you can try reversing the motion and swing the rope from front to back. Or you can try going faster and whipping the rope under your feet for two revolutions before you land.

You can also travel as you jump, no reason to stay in one spot. Pretend you're hurtling over obstacles in pursuit of fleeing quarry or something. Have some fun!

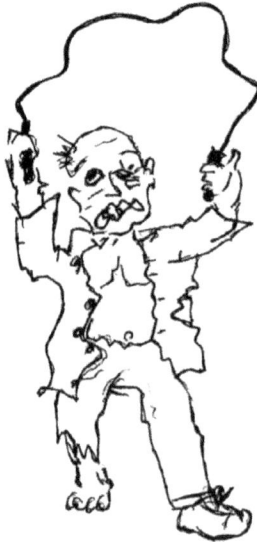

The Exercises

The Squat

Squats are the quintessential quadriceps builder, and work your hips, butt, hamstrings, and calves as well. All that lower body strength will help you launch victims clean off the ground with greater ease when you tackle them.

From a standing position, you sit back/squat down until your thighs are parallel to the floor, with your upper back straight and your lower back slightly arched. In a proper squat, be sure to sit back – do not allow your knees to move farther forward than your toes.

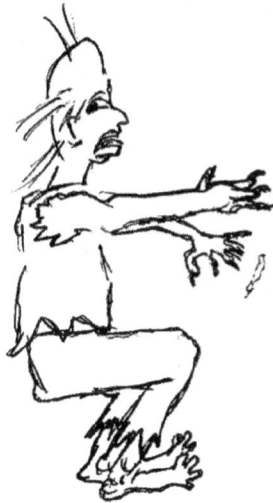

If the Squats get too easy with no weight, add a backpack with some books or rocks in it, then fire away. You may want to stand in front of a couch or a chair, to catch yourself if you pitch backward. If you do collapse in a heap, just scramble back up and try again. Once you feel fatigue set in after a number of reps, conclude the Squat workout for now. Do these every third day.

The Windmill

The Windmill is one of those exercises often considered out of style, both by the living and Zombie communities. How unfortunate. Windmills are excellent for working a large percentage of your body at once, with special emphasis on the lower back and the hamstrings. This motion will help you grab morsels from the ground, maintain your ability to bend and straighten back up with vigor, apprehend victims already at your feet, and put a spring in your step. So let's do some Windmills.

Stand with feet shoulder-width apart, arms straight out to the sides. Twist and bend at the waist while reaching your right hand down to your left foot, return to starting position. Repeat with left hand reaching down to your right foot. Keep going until you start to feel exhausted. Do these every third day, no more, as your hamstrings could end up quite sore otherwise. Don't want to be losing a leg any sooner than need be, after all.

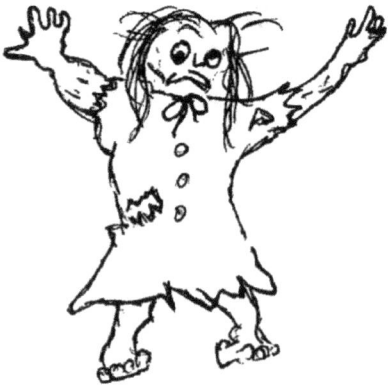

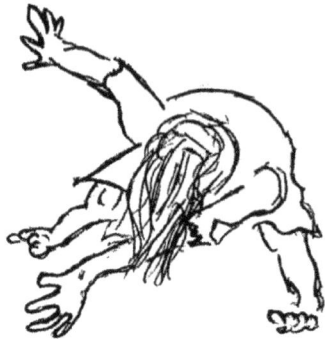

Calf Raise

Every type of stepping motion you do will be improved with the strengthening of your calf muscles. Whether maneuvering down an incline, climbing stairs, attempting a lurching run, or standing your ground and battling an intended victim, strong calves will solidify your base and propel you with authority. You'll be able to walk with a swagger, once you put some extra power in your stagger!

As the name implies, doing repetitions with the Calf Raise works your calves, the muscles on the back of your lower legs. As you do them, you can hold dumbbells or other appropriate weights – rocks from the rubble, old boards scattered on the ground, even discarded sections of other Zombies – to increase resistance and make this portion of your workout more effective. Pictured is an exerciser holding a skull, which is just one type of object you can use as a weight. Of course, when just starting out, you can simply do the calf raises with bodyweight only.

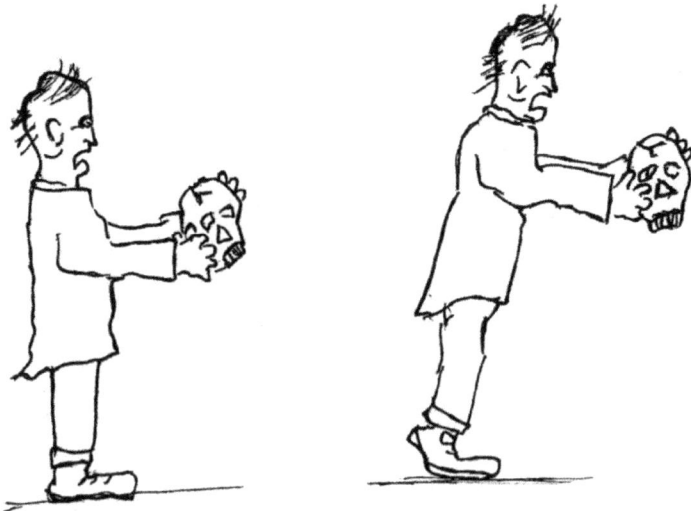

From a standing position, keep your knees straight and rise up on your toes as high as possible. Hold the flexion for a full second. As you get better with this motion, do them one leg at a time if using no weight.

Work the Calf Raise until exhaustion, then stop. That's one set. Work up to three or four sets over time; do them every other day.

As you execute the reps, make sure to not fall forward, especially if you often flail for long periods of time while getting back to your feet. Focus.

Pushup

Dedicate your efforts to the Pushup, and realize the following payoff: when your living adversaries shove you, you'll be able to shove them back with greater force. Then hopefully clutch them with more authority for the harvest. And that's just a couple of the benefits a Pushup routine provides. Let's get started.

The Pushup is the classic and great all-around upper body builder. You can perform this exercise with your legs extended straight behind you, or with bent knees resting on the floor. If you need your knees down on the floor, it's all good. That's not "cheating." That modified method is still a great strength builder. It's just a different form than the knees up, straight body position.

Keep hands level with your shoulders; how far out from the shoulders will determine which shoulder muscles get the most focus. Closer together emphasizes your triceps, further out focuses on the front of your shoulders. All hand positions will still allow the chest to be worked as you complete the Pushups. Do as many as you can consecutively, and that's one set. See if you can't add a second or third set over time.

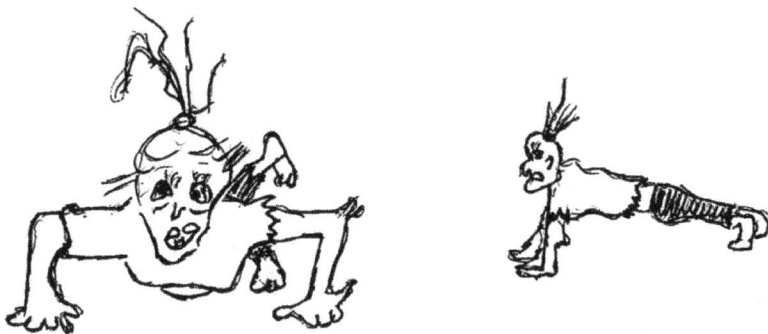

Get strong and efficient at the Pushup motion. Doing so almost assures you'll be able to pop back up to your feet with ease after those times that you end up on the ground. As the days wear on, collapsing into the dirt may occur with greater frequency for a variety of reasons. Not the least of which being the decayed lower body that most Zombies have to face eventually. So be strong in the areas where you can. Do your Pushups.

Front Raise

This awesome exercise works the shoulder muscles, mainly the side deltoids. These are important muscles to keep strong for fending off counterattacks from your intended victims, and for making your backhand blows really count when you strike them. Strong shoulders are also important when carrying leftovers.

Hold a dumbbell or other appropriate weight – a discarded backpack filled with some rocks, a large bone, etc. – in each hand, resting it in front of your thighs, palms facing your body and elbows slightly bent. Raise the weight up to eye level, keeping the arm relatively straight. Hold for 1-2 seconds and lower that arm. That's one repetition. Do as many Front Raises as you can until you feel your muscles tire. Switch the weight to the other hand (if you still have both hands) and raise that other arm in the same manner.

Just one set with each arm should do the trick per workout; do these every other or every third day.

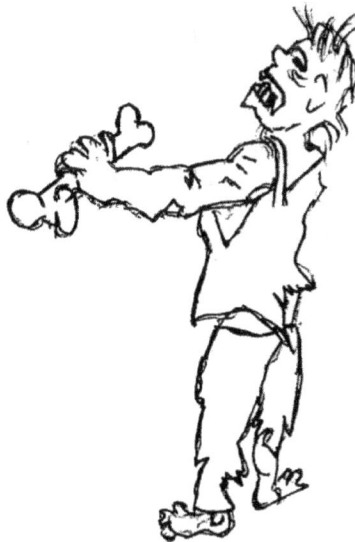

Biceps Curl

Biceps strength is especially valuable when you're part of a feeding frenzy, as it assists in powerful scooping motions. Your main adversaries are your prey, of course, but why let fellow Zombies out-compete you? The Biceps Curl will give you that extra edge during group frenzies, helping you to get your share.

To complete a Biceps Curl, use your biceps to curl, or raise in a semi-circle, a dumbbell (or barbell if using both hands at once) from your hips up to chest level. Lower to complete one repetition. Repeat until you feel your biceps begin to tire. That's one set, and that should be all you need in a given workout. Do the Biceps Curl every other or every third day.

Note: one cool trick for an incentive is to use a bone with some meat still on it, and curl it to your mouth, take just a small nibble, then lower it back down. That's one repetition; curl it up again for another taste. Use that method, and this section of your workout will be done before you know it. Incentives rock!

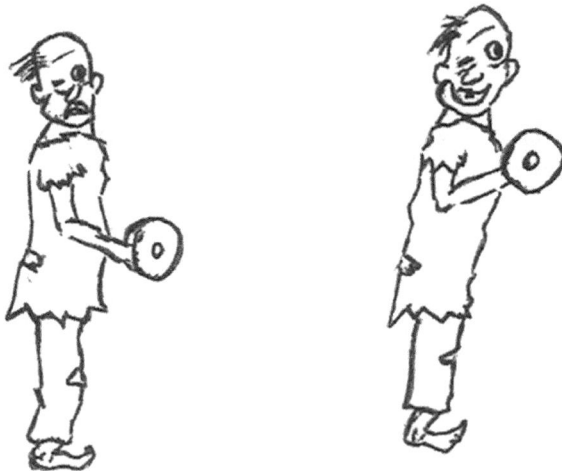

Weight-Assisted Step-Ups

Remember when you were one of the living? You were scampering around, trying to not get grabbed by one of your current colleagues in the Zombie community. It's a safe bet that when the pressure was really on, and they almost had you, to get away you ran in a key direction. *Up*. Up a hill, up a staircase. And the Zombies were left behind.

Why? Because Zombies are terrible at climbing stairs and hills. And, as you might know, you now *are* a Zombie. And how's that climbing hills and staircases thing working out for you? Not so well?

Rectify the dilemma with some Weight-assisted Step-ups. The motion will be like climbing steps, usually two at a time, but you'll add some weight to increase effectiveness. Once you go back to climbing hills and stairs with no extra resistance, you won't believe the improvement you'll have made.

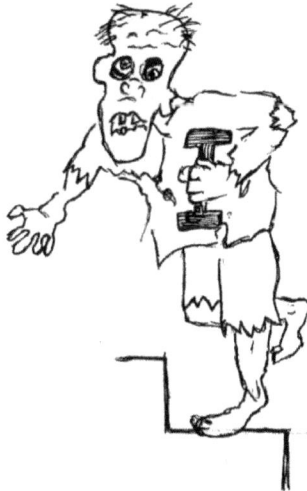

To do the motion, hold a weight in your hand, such as a dumbbell, a victim's filled backpack, a heavy brick, or a large bone. At a flight of steps, just step up like you normally would. Go two stairs at a time if possible. Lower yourself back down, then quickly step back up. Repeat over and over until you feel a burn; that concludes the set. Remember to lead with alternating legs to work them both, if they both still function. Do this routine every other day.

Cable (or Sapling) Crossover

Another great exercise for your upper body. The Crossover focuses on the chest muscles, and your core muscles will get in on the action as well.

Use a cable and pulley system in an abandoned gymnasium if you can find one. Or maybe stumble onto an old construction site where some pulleys are still in place. Get creative and put a piece of twine through the pulley and tie a brick or block on the other end perhaps.

If nothing like a cable and pulley system is around, see if you can't find a flexible, small tree in the area; a tender little sapling is ideal. Then grab one of the slender branches and twist it as if it's a weighted cable.

To perform the Crossover motion, grab the cable or branch, and move the resistance down and across your body. Basically, a motion from your shoulder area over to your opposite hip is the idea. Move the resistance, hold it in the finished position for a second, then relax back to the starting position. Do the exercise until exhausted, then wrap it up for that side. Repeat the exercise using the opposite hand. Do a set of Crossovers every third day.

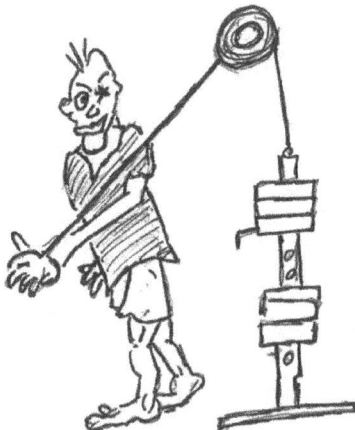

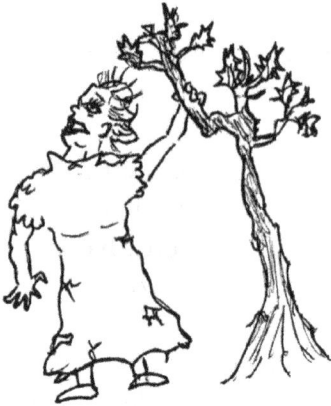

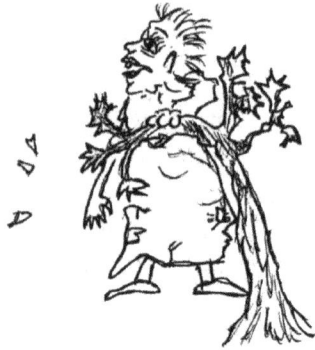

If using a sapling for this exercise, make sure it is flexible enough to handle the range of motion. No need to leave extra destruction in your path. Save it for the victims.

Lateral Raise

Similar to the Front Raise, the Lateral Raise exercise works the shoulder muscles, in other words the deltoids.

Carrying loads of meat and bone requires sturdy shoulders. The ability to lug heavy quantities will help when you're saving some for later. And the strength given by the Lateral Raise motion will make your arm waving and flailing less exhausting. Acquire more purposeful arm swings and you'll soon be staggering around with style. Here's how to complete a proper Lateral Raise.

Hold a dumbbell in each hand down by your sides, with elbows slightly bent. Raise the weights straight up away from your sides to approximately shoulder level. Keep the arms relatively straight, with just that slight elbow bend. Lower to complete one repetition. Repeat until you feel exhaustion setting in; that completes one set. Move on to the next exercise. Do the Lateral Raise every other or every third day.

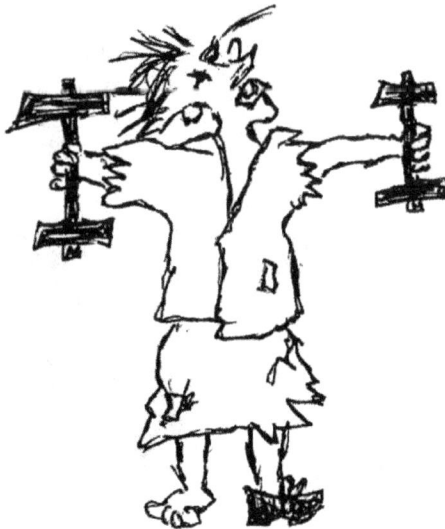

Deadlift

What exercise could be more fitting for members of the undead community? Even the name of the motion, the *Deadlift,* sets the tone for the most intrepid of Zombies enjoying an undead life.

The Deadlift motion is simple to master, and provides you with several benefits. After sticking to a regular program including Deadlifts, here are just a few actions you'll be able to perform with greater ease:

- Flipping over bodies to select the most valuable portions.

- Opening trapdoors where victims may be hiding underground.

- Yanking weapons away from fallen victims.

- Picking up and carrying carcasses.

That's a pretty decent payoff for doing such a simple motion, don't you think? Here's how to execute the Deadlift:

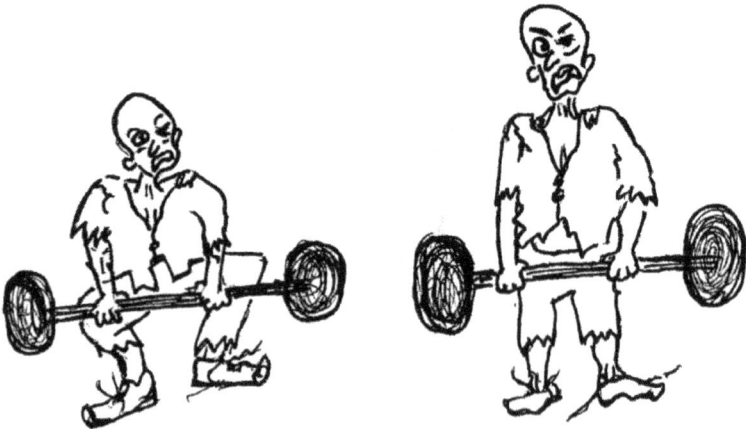

Crouch down next to the barbell, and grip the bar with hands about shoulder width apart. Keep your back relatively straight, and look up. Then simply straighten your back, bring your hips forward, and heave the barbell from the ground as you stand up. Hold the bar for a couple of seconds, then lower the bar to the ground. Or just let it drop with a slam; this is the wild, wild world of the post-apocalypse, after all. The clanking slam helps set the tone of your ferocious new fitness! Aim the dropping barbell out away from your feet.

Repeat the motion a time or two, then call it quits on the Deadlift for the day. Do the Deadlift every other or every third day.

Overhead Press

Having trouble lifting bones and skulls overhead in victory? This exercise is sure to help you solve that issue. The Overhead Press works your shoulder muscles, triceps, and tests your midsection stability. What's more, if you vanquish any foes that previously made fun of you, this is a nice way to prepare for picking them up overhead and flinging them. A very Alpha Zombie move.

To begin the Overhead Press, heft the barbell or other weight from the ground (see the Deadlift chapter for proper lifting), and rest it at the top of your chest. Flex your knees a little, then straighten them and pop the weight upward. Then just extend your arms, duck your head under, and hold the bar in place for a moment. That's one repetition.

If you get stuck on the last rep, due to either lack of enthusiasm or impending decay, try to picture your prey. Especially any who have recently eluded you, leaving you hungry and embarrassed. This should empower you for that final repetition. Let out a loud moan and power up that bar.

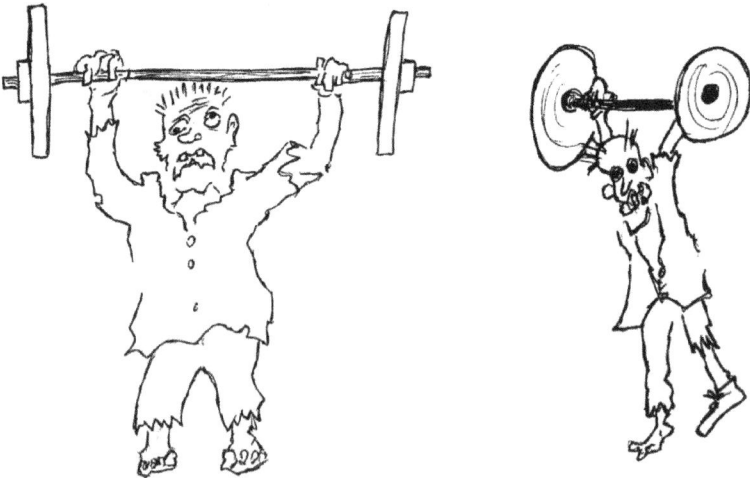

After a vigorous set with one hard last repetition as described, you may feel weakness setting in. That's a good time to place the weight back on the ground until next time. That concludes your set. Don't overdo the reps here, or your arms and shoulders could give out and the barbell or other weight could smack down on your already delicate head and knock you senseless. Use caution when performing the Overhead Press.

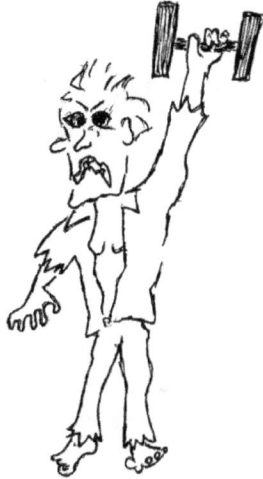

Note: The Overhead Press done one arm at a time is a great approach as well. Bones, rocks, dumbbells, and metal scraps lying on the ground are all ideal for doing a one-armed Overhead Press.

Pullup

Ever have prey climb a tree to escape you? Or up to the top of a high fence, from where they then drop safely to the other side of that barrier? Happens to Zombies all the time, leaving them deflated and unfulfilled. Is there a way to improve upon this shortcoming? Yes: perform the Pullup.

Do enough Pullups, and the next time some arrogant member of the living scrambles up and over a protective boundary, thinking safety has been achieved, you'll be able to go after them with full energy. They think they are safe, but if you've regularly worked on your Pullups...forget about it. You can now catch them.

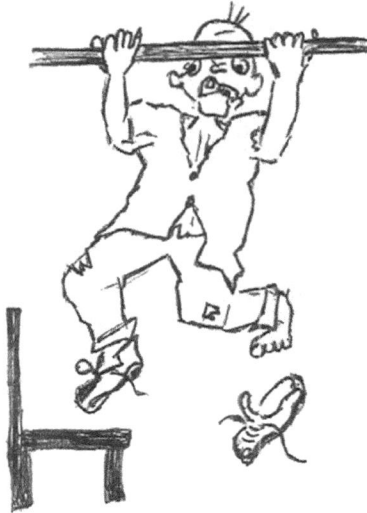

You'll need a Pullup bar installed in a doorjamb for Pullups. As an alternative, find a sturdy branch or an old pipe suspended from the ground amidst the rubble. Reach up and grab the bar, with palms facing away, or facing toward you, it doesn't matter. You ideally will grip the bar both ways on different sets. Pull yourself on up, and see if you can bring your chin to the bar. If you can't, and many Zombies at first can't, add a little jump to start your upward movement. If you still can't complete the motion, just hold the flexed position of your arms a couple of seconds. Do this flexion several times for one set. That in itself is a tremendous workout.

Do some Pullups every third day; eventually you'll get there. And then you'll be able to get to those that climb up and away from you.

Lunge

Whether you're trying to dive in and capture your prey, or just get under their guard during a confrontation, the ability to lunge and tackle is the name of the game. The Lunge exercise done regularly will help with these efforts.

The Lunge works your rump, hips, the entirety of your upper legs, and your lower legs to a lesser extent.

To start, step forward with one foot into a split stance...in other words, where the forward foot plants in front of you and your back foot props up on its ball and toes. Push your hips back and bend your knees to lower down; in other words, basically drop into the lunge. Your back knee lowers to within a few inches of the floor. Be cautious about hitting the floor forcefully with your back knee...ouch! Do not push your front knee forward; instead, focus on the downward motion of the lunge.

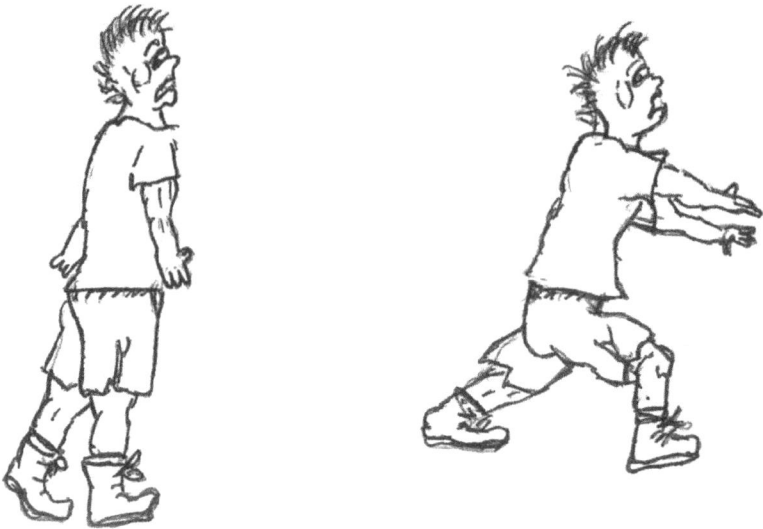

If you collapse during the first few tries, just sway and lurch back up to your feet, and give the Lunge another try. You'll get it with some practice.

When you feel soreness set in on the muscles involved, switch to work the other leg. When you feel soreness set in for that leg, stop and rest a minute or two. Maybe think of prey evading you as you rest, to psych yourself for set number two. Once rested, repeat the same motion for each leg, and when rest is needed again, conclude the Lunge for today. After two days of rest, repeat the workout.

The Double-Crunch

Zombies often experience their first full-body collapse due to a weak midsection; sometimes they never recover. Unable to keep feeding, they just lie there and decay. Yuck! Don't let it happen to you.

The Double-Crunch is a great exercise for your midsection, namely your abdominals, or abs for short. To start, lie flat on your back with your knees bent and your feet flat on the floor; loosely place your hands behind your head or cross your arms over your chest. Tighten your abs as you breathe out and lift your shoulders off the floor; at the same time, pull your knees towards your head. Bring head and knees as close together as you can. Then lower to the starting position to complete one repetition.

Crank them out until you feel exhaustion setting in, then rest. That concludes your Double-Crunch workout. Do these every third day.

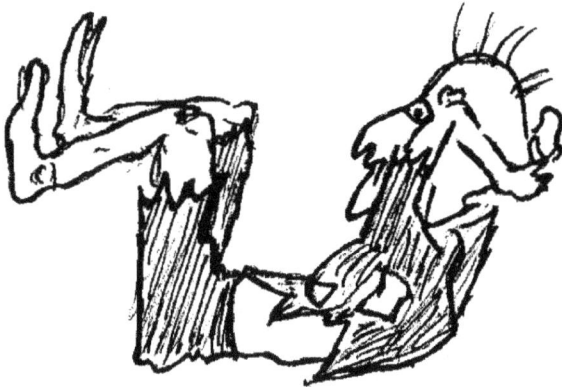

The Plank

As previously mentioned, after tumbling to the ground, many Zombie citizens experience trouble getting back to their feet. If this describes you, here's a fine exercise to help you address this problem and get back up and at 'em. Like the Double-Crunch on the previous page the Plank strengthens the muscles of your lower back, abdominals, and sides, the combination of which is often referred to as your "core." A solid core is crucial for the quickest scramble possible from a fallen-down position to the back-in-action position.

Start by lying face down and propping yourself up on your forearms. Keep your elbows directly below your shoulders. Your legs should be straight, and your feet less than shoulder-width apart. Push your hips off the ground by engaging your hip and abdominal muscles until your body is in a straight line; brace yourself with your forearms. Ensure your head is in line with your neutral spine.

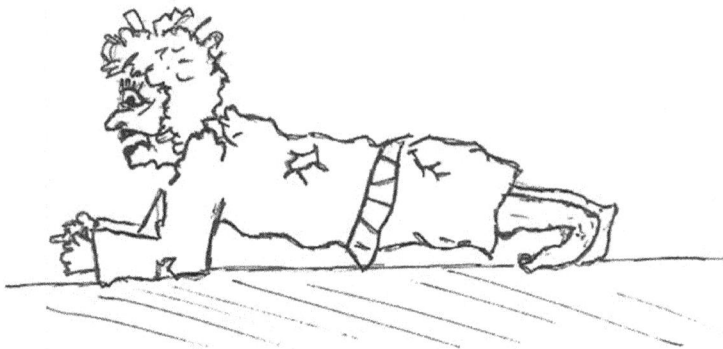

See if you can hold the position for 10 seconds or so. If 10 seconds becomes easy, go for about 20. Then rest; that's it for Plank action for the day. Try to do the Plank every third day or so.

Important tips: Keep your abdominals tight while performing the Plank, and do not let your hips sag to the floor. Also, your head and neck should be in line with your spine.

For additional benefit, practice popping your jaws while in the flexed position, to keep that tenacious edge. Plus, the jaw-popping provides an extra benefit: you may some day feed while in this position; do the Plank and you'll arrive for the feast prepared.

Complementary Activities

Hill Walking

Hill walking can make your thighs burn and calves ache, and you'll realize all those Squats and Step-ups have a real-life purpose. Or real-undead purpose. Or something. Strength training is not only for nice-looking muscles, but also to help you venture out into the world and then help you return with some sustenance: i.e., some vanquished prey.

Plan the shortest hill walk possible to become familiar with the feel of the endeavor. Increase the distance and size of hill selected gradually. Put in a hill walk every other day or so.

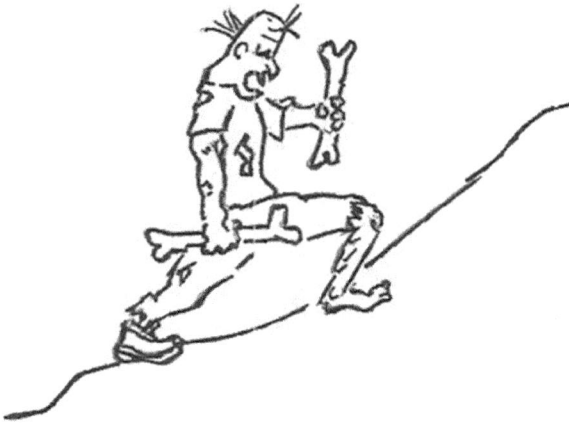

Punch It Out

Here's a great all-around exercise endeavor that in addition provides realistic application for fighting your battles – and winning. What could be more natural, fulfilling, and tension-relieving than doing an exercise where you can simulate busting heads, overwhelming your adversaries with unquestionable force, and being able to do this without being burdened by any expensive or unwieldy equipment. As a matter of fact, the enemy doesn't even have to be there...you can just pretend. You're almost guaranteed to win.

The exercise: the Punching workout.

Not only will this work pretty much your entire upper body, it's also a great way to release the frustrations caused by the daily grind. The failures...the frustrations...the near-misses...the never-ending hunger. *Arrgghh! Heeee-yaaaa!!*

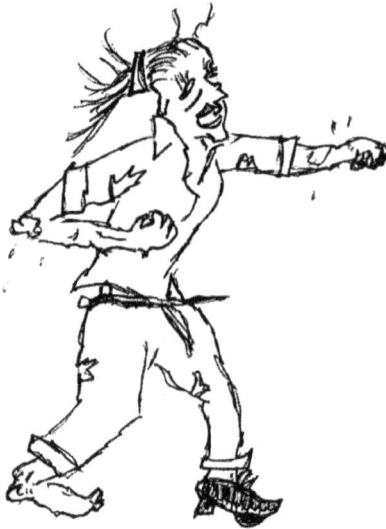

OK, back to the Punching workout. Some Zombies have chosen to do this with a formal approach, using traditional martial arts striking methods like those done in Tae Kwon Do.

Others have went with good old-fashioned boxing movements. Both ways are ideal.

And be aware, there is a third, and simpler, way to do the Punching workout: crazy swinging! Use overhand swings, roundhouse punches, uppercuts, jabs, straight lefts and rights from a square stance, you name it. Just go berserk. Do that with enough insanity in view of your fellow Zombies, and I assure you, few will try to steal your leftover scraps.

After about 30 seconds or so, call it quits for the day. Do the Punching workout every third day or so.

Just Dance!

Do it for joy, do it to blow off steam, do it out of rage...whatever the reason, lose your inhibitions, cut yourself loose, and just dance!

Not only is dancing a great way to work on your rhythm, it also makes for a wonderful workout. You'll keep muscles nice and twitchy for the chase, and stave off the limpness of the undead at the same time.

Plus, here is a perfect time to let out your weirdest, most haunted wails and squeals; no one will question it if dancing is taking place! So go ahead: get your blood pumping, limbs shaking, and hips wiggling (just not too hard, lest some body parts go flying).

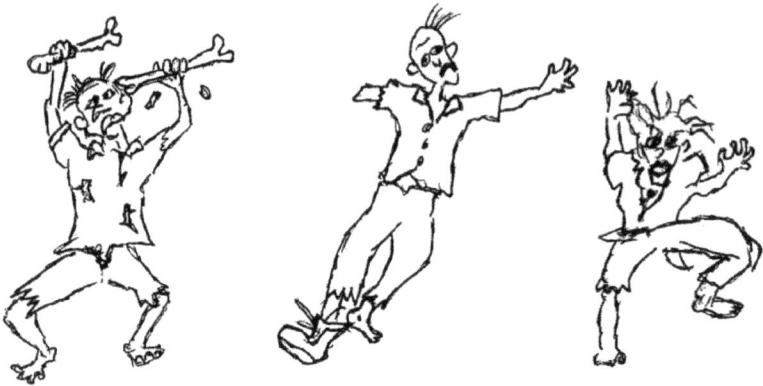

Stretches

Hamstring Stretch

Flexible muscles will make your workout more effective and safe. And when it comes to important areas to have limber, few spots on your body are as crucial as your hamstrings. Tight hamstrings can be tough to live with...even for the non-living. Not only do inflexible hamstrings put these long, strong muscles in the back of your thighs themselves at risk, above and beyond normal Zombie decay, but they also cause undue tension on other body parts. The most publicized by-product of stiff hamstrings is the extra wear and tear they cause on the lower back.

Developing hamstring flexibility is quite beneficial to your entire body. It assists in ease of movement in just about every motion your body can perform, during both your exercise routines and your daily tasks of grabbing and subduing quarry. And it feels good, almost a relief, when tight hamstrings get good and loosened up. A number of good hamstring stretches are out there, and here's one that is effective, safe, and somewhat relaxing.

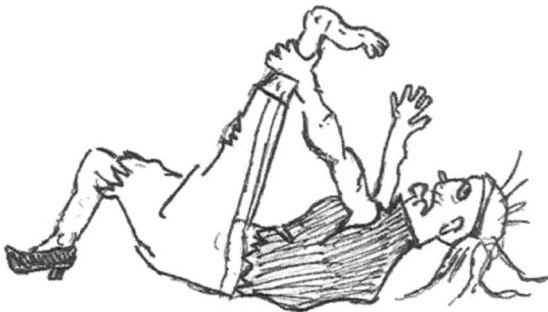

While on your back, raise one leg, keeping it bent at the knee just a bit; with one or both hands, hold the leg behind the knee (or closer to the ankle if you have the flexibility), and slowly, gently extend your leg. This will stretch the hamstring area. Expect the hamstring to be a little tight if you have not stretched it regularly since your transition. Flexing your foot while stretching the hamstring will extend the stretch to your calf area as well.

A slight variation to this procedure is to wrap a towel around the center of your foot, versus holding your leg with your hands. Pull carefully on the towel as you extend your leg, stopping and holding the position once you feel a stretch begin.

Hold the stretch for about 10-20 seconds, and repeat the process once or twice. Switch legs to reap the same benefits for your other leg.

If you currently have exceptional flexibility from living in an already-dead body, make sure not to stretch too far...especially not to the point of contortions or anything. You want to keep those remaining joints and tissues intact as best possible.

Overhead Side Stretch

For the overhead stretch, you'll simply be reaching up and over. This all-around useful stretch will stretch your upper back and shoulders.

Do this gently at first; your fellow Zombies have been known from time to time to tear a shoulder or side muscle when doing this too abruptly. Some have even had entire arms fall off. Of course, if you live long enough as one of the undead, body parts are going to separate and go by the wayside. But let's not rush things. Proceed with care.

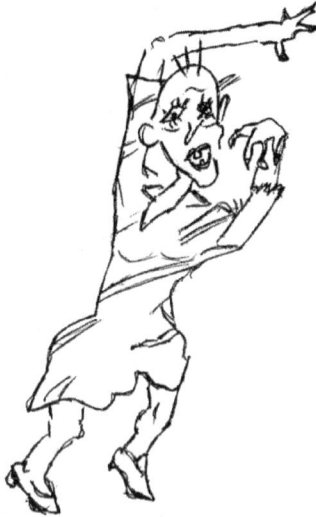

Standing straight, with feet approximately shoulder width apart, reach up with your right arm and lean towards your left side. Use that extended arm as a lever to incorporate a good stretch; the further you reach, the more fully you will stretch. For balance, feel free to hold onto a chair or a section of wasteland rubble with your left hand.

Once you feel the stretch take place, go no further. Hold the stretch for 10-20 seconds. Rest a moment, and repeat. Then reverse directions and perform the stretch for your left side.

To Your Health

Eat Right

An important thing to remember in your Zombie fitness endeavors is that nutrition plays a critical part. As if you didn't already know it, right? Hunger haunts your every staggering moment, those hours and hours filled with aimless groaning and wandering, the urge to feast dominating your endless ordeal as you search for fresh victims. It's a tough way to exist.

But there are solutions to fill the gaps and address the emptiness of the despair that Zombies know all too well. To make ends meet nutritionally, try to follow these four guiding principles:

- **Drink plenty of water.**
  Whether consuming adequate amounts of water helps a Zombie or not, nobody knows. But it will stave off hunger, and your primitive, deteriorating brain just might recognize it as the fresh intake of a victim. Plus, always remember: you may feel hungry, but maybe you're really just thirsty.

- **Avoid hydrogenated fats.**
  Commonly referred to as "trans fats," this form of fat is a product of a natural substance that had, for the sake of shelf life, been altered by humankind into an artificial paste; one not recognized by the Zombie body as a food at all...and then processed into products that the commercial food industry served people to eat, way back when there was civilization. Oh yum. Trans fats are overwhelmingly bad news, for both satisfaction and for overall Zombie fitness.

Healthy, naturally-occurring fats, as opposed to the aforementioned trans fats, can be one of your best allies in the Zombie fitness lifestyle. And have no fear; intake of fat for a Zombie will rarely be "artery clogging." On the contrary, plenty of research indicates healthful side effects of some fat in your diet, including saturated fat. Humankind had consumed fat, and plenty of it, for thousands of years. You're now beyond your human phase of life, but some remnants of evolution still gurgle inside of you; what is good for a human will often be good for you the Zombie too.

So regarding fat intake, when tearing into old cans and jars you might find in the food larders of vacant houses and buildings, as a rule avoid hydrogenated fat and eat natural fat.

- Bone up for top health.

Whatever happened to the lust for bones? In the Zombie community, the emphasis lately seems to be brains, brains, brains. But a pile of bones can represent some stellar nutrition, from both the bone itself and the marrow inside of it. Plus, most of your Zombie cohorts will discard the bones of victims, and go off searching for more choice morsels. There's your chance!

When you have a food source secured, make the best of it and eat those bones. When others leave bones behind, scavenge them. Your system will thank you for it.

- Brains ain't everything.

We just discussed a similar thought above, but it bears repeating. Embrace your omnivore side. Face it: most Zombies aren't in a position to be choosy. Take advantage of whatever calorie sources you can find.

As a Zombie, brains may be like catnip to you; fat satiates you; protein keeps your strength up and your muscles from deteriorating any faster than they already are. But what about plant sources? We recommend that you occasionally ingest plant material if possible. If you come across a fruit source, such as an old apple orchard, a thorny raspberry bush, or maybe a patch of wild strawberries, dig in. The fruit taste may be disagreeable at first, but keep in mind, it's all about calories. You need the energy supply.

The same applies to vegetables, whether you find a canned supply you can smash open, or an abandoned farm area where some plants still flourish. Pick and eat whatever you can. That applies to patches of weeds too, if nothing else is available. Stuff them in your gaping mouth, chew them up, and don't complain. If it makes it any easier, pretend it's a vanquished victim you're eating.

These four cornerstones for eating should help you make ends meet when prey sources are scarce. Be ready to adjust and do what works best for you. It's possible to enjoy plenty of flexibility in an individualized program and secure lots of plentiful, nutritious foods, other than counting completely on brains and holding out forever for them.

In short, keep your options open, stay hydrated, and eat whatever presents itself. *Bon Appetit!*

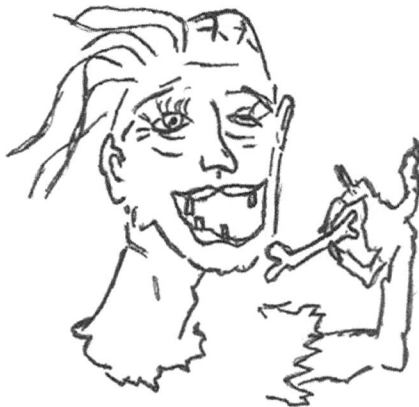

Get Plenty of Rest

Sleep is important for the fitness-minded Zombie, as this is the time when your body repairs itself, digests your devoured food, and prepares for the next hunting conquest.

After a few consecutive nights of poor sleep you may find yourself with an out-of-control appetite; this is mostly because sleep deprivation causes the hormones which regulate your appetite to get thrown out of whack.

Researchers have found that significant changes in the levels of the hormones *ghrelin* and *leptin* occur when you get less than 5 hours of sleep. Lack of sleep increases ghrelin and decreases leptin from their normal levels. This sensitive hormone balance helps control your appetite. Ghrelin is used to whet your appetite; if its level is excessive, your appetite will be excessive as well. As if acquiring enough food for a Zombie wasn't challenge enough!

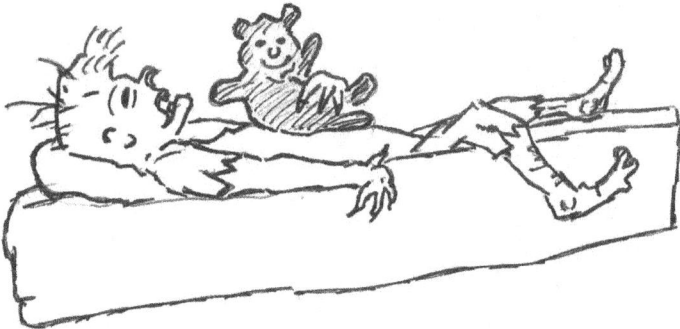

Long before the Zombie Apocalypse, a University of Chicago study found that getting an average of just 6.5 hours of sleep each night can be detrimental to the mind and body. Most Zombies need more than 6.5 hours of sleep, based on such studies. The National Sleep Foundation in the past recommended 7-9 hours of sleep each night. And despite doubters and myths surrounding the taking of naps, sleep specialists generally agree that naps do indeed help to correct the effects of sleep deprivation. Otherwise, Zombies wouldn't naturally take them.

Do what you can to get enough sleep. Make it a priority. In your past life, plenty of rest and deep sleep would help you feel fully alive. Now things are different, but you can achieve a similar positive effect from adequate sleep. Get enough shut-eye and you'll be able to stalk victims while feeling energetic and fully undead. Undead, yet refreshed.

Final Words

Time to seize the new dawn!

Fit to be fed. Feels good, doesn't it?

Remember back when the Zombie Fitness regimen seemed insurmountable? So much to learn, and considering your steady decay, so little time in which to learn it. But you came, you saw, you devoured. You did it. Now you are the workout routine's master.

I know, I know. Many of the old problems still remain. The prey you seek remain elusive. They maneuver through their secret hideouts, staying hidden. They sprint away from you in the streets, showing their agility and leaving you tottering on the edge. It can feel futile sometimes.

Plus, maintaining a training schedule for optimal fitness is not always easy. At times you may need to put in extra time on the hunt. At other moments, you may need to rest. Rest is indeed important, and we thus covered it previously. But you can only rest so much; just keep lying there like a member of the truly dead and you'll never end up well-fed and fulfilled. You have to rest a little, then train a lot and hunt a lot.

And if you're like most Zombies, you may not always feel like doing either. But you must. Drop the excuses. Had a long, hard week chasing your victims down? Hearing the other Zombies murmur about you regarding your new fitness routine? Lost another body part? Regardless of any of these external factors, you should still push on and persevere, bringing your 'A' game to both the hunt and the workouts. Do it or stay forever hungry.

Attitude. That's what it's all about. Bask in your whole new level of fitness; rejoice in the fresh awakening. A new dawn, and a new you. Well, maybe you'll still flake apart now and then, but still. Even little improvements are a step forward.

And keep this in mind: the powers that be chose only certain individuals to carry on and on in the post-apocalypse. One of those chosen was *you*. After knowing you've been gifted with this special calling, can you allow yourself to lumber around and mope? Would you even want to? That grunt you just gave sounded like a no.

So make the choice to be tenacious. Decide to be a winner. Feel the new strength coursing through your aging tissues. Know that those prized members of the prey community, those tempting morsels, are hiding and scampering out there like jumpy jitterbugs. They're yours for the taking. So get ahold of yourself, and decide.

Remember who you've become; remember what it took to get here. The moans, the groans, the early frustrations. The newly discovered glee. After embracing and completing the coursework in the Zombie Fitness program, you've become a member of the Zombie elite; start acting like it. Choose greatness. Maintain your newfound Zombie fitness, and proceed to use it.

Then look alive, and stumble forth to seize your prey.

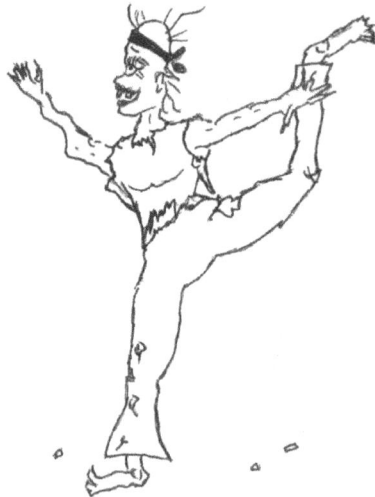

Zombie Fitness Manual   45

About the Author

P. J. Hafner has been involved in fitness and conditioning for over 30 years, including 15 years in wrestling and martial arts, numerous hikes all over North America and Europe, and running in over 100 races. Like a man possessed, he's done enough training to sometimes feel like one of the undead.

Although a St. Paul, Minnesota native, the last several years have found Hafner living all over the U.S., moving around so much you'd almost think he was being chased by the intended audience of this manual.

This is his first Zombie self-help book.

www.ingramcontent.com/pod-product-compliance
Lightning Source LLC
Chambersburg PA
CBHW060655280326
41933CB00012B/2187